The Food Lord

ABC Book of Superfoods

Antonio Ford

The Food Lord

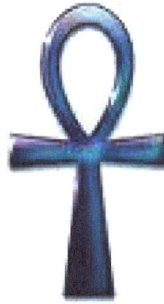

ABC Book of

Superfoods

By Antonio Ford

The Food Lord ABC Book of Superfoods
Copyright © 2016 by Antonio Ford

ISBN-13:978-0-9971609-2-5

ISBN-10:0-9971609-2-6

Go to www.cookingwiththefoodlord.info to buy additional copies.

Contact Antonio Ford, The Food Lord, at **aford_1967@yahoo.com**

I'd like to dedicate this powerful book to my wife Danielle Ford for doing a wonderful job on making this work come to life.

To my son and daughter Seven and Serenity.

WHO MOTIVATE ME REGULARLY!

I'd like to thank all my friends, family, and my Brussel Sprouts who have always encouraged me to write.

When we have this type of truth around you, It changes things, I intend on making a difference with food and my words

ONE BITE AT A TIME

ANTONIO FORD

AKA

THE FOOD LORD

A

Acai Berries

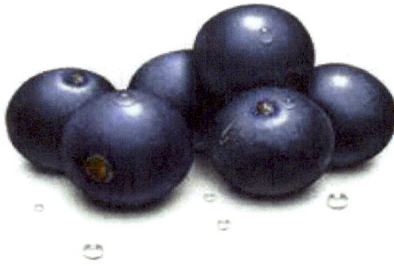

Known as the **"Beauty Berry"**

B

Brussel Sprouts

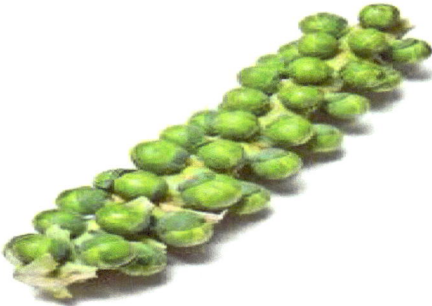

Brussel Sprouts look like "miniature cabbages."

C

Cherries

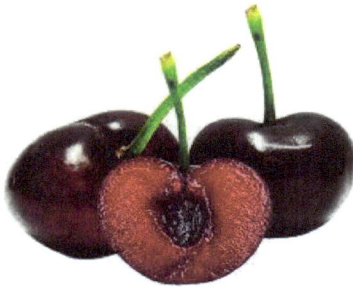

The **cherry** fruit is part of the Rosaceae family which also includes almonds, peaches, apricots, and plums.

D

Dragon Fruit

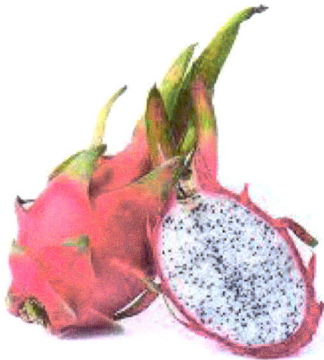

"Dragon Fruits" real name is "Pitaya." It refers to fruit of the genus Hylocereus.

E

Eggplant

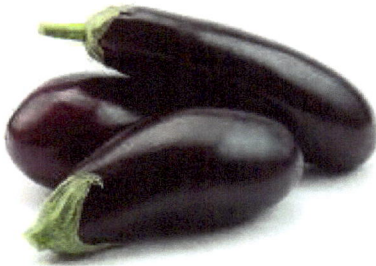

Eggplant, or Aubergine, is a species of nightshade grown for its edible fruit. The eggplant is extremely high in fiber.

F

Fig

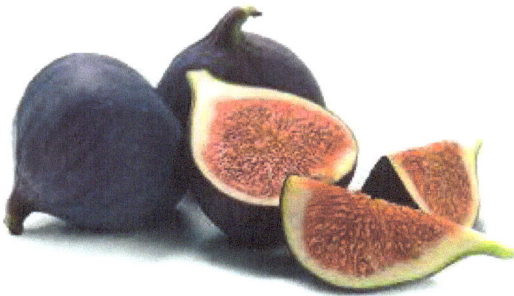

The **fig** tree is a symbol of abundance, fertility, and sweetness.

G

Grapes

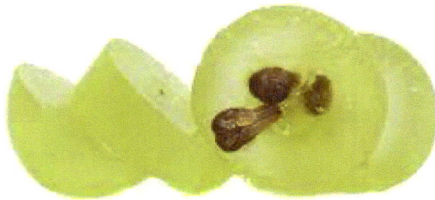

Anti-Aging property of **grapes** is proved by many researches. Its constitution of around 20 popular anti-oxidants makes it the most sought after beautifying product.

H

Honey

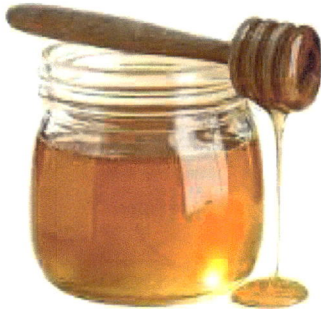

Honey is a sweet food made by bees foraging nectar from flowers.

I

Indian Pea

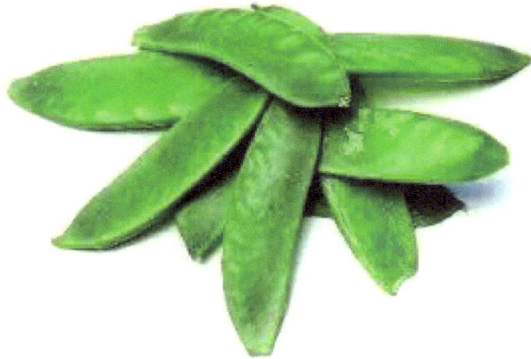

Indian Peas are green because they are harvested when not fully mature.

J

Juniper Berries

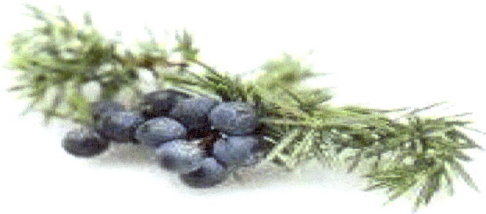

A **juniper berry** is the female seed cone produced by
the various species of junipers.

K

Kale

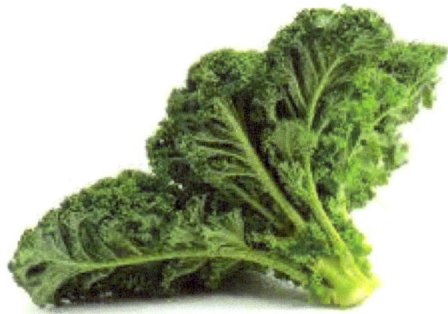

1 cup of raw **kale** has just 33 calories yet contains 684% of vitamin K, 134% of vitamin C, 206% of Vitamin A plus iron, folate, omega-3s, magnesium, calcium, iron, fiber, and 2 grams of protein.

L

Lentils

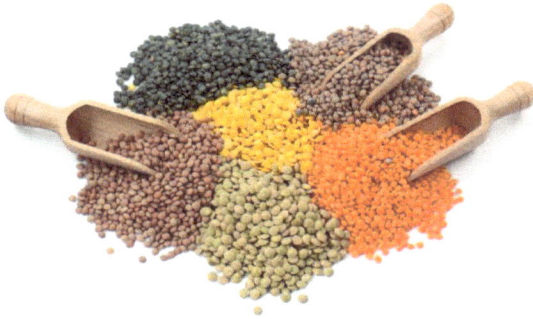

One cup of **lentils** provides almost half your daily recommended intake of manganese.

M

Mushrooms

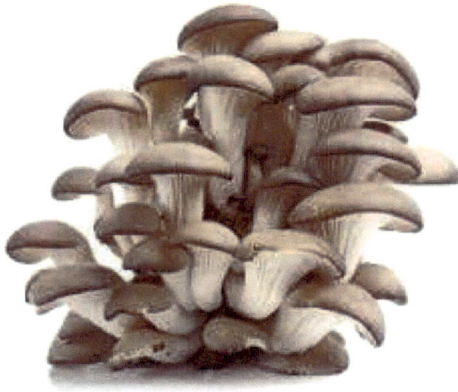

Mushrooms are made up of around 90% water. Mushrooms are a fungus, and unlike plants, mushrooms do not require sunlight to make energy for themselves.

N

Nutmeg

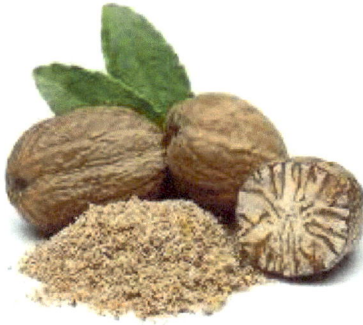

Whole **nutmeg** keeps almost indefinitely stored in airtight containers, but ground nutmeg loses its flavor very quick.

O

Oranges

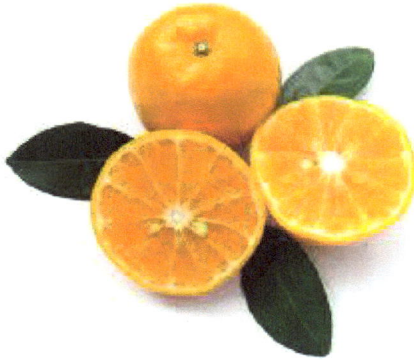

Around 85% of all **oranges** produced are used for juice.

P

Pomegranate

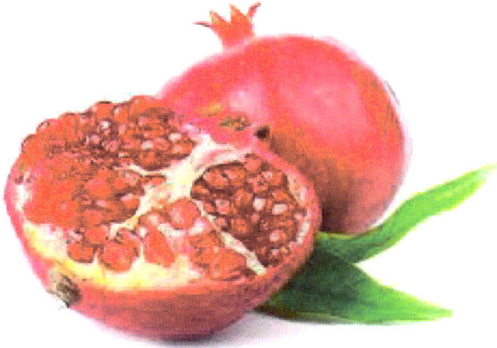

Pomegranates grown in the United States are typically in season from September to December.

Q

Quince

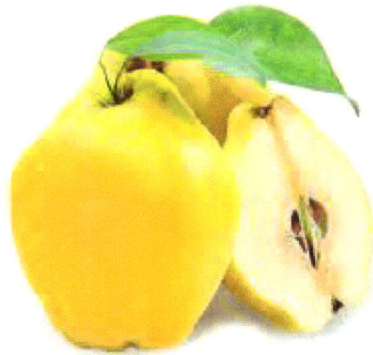

Quince is deciduous tree that belongs to the family of roses.

R

Raspberries

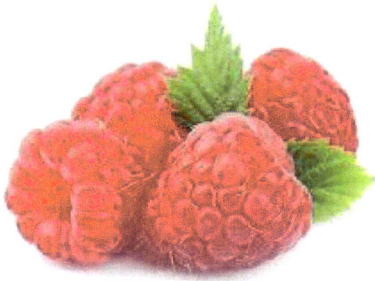

The word **"raspberry"** seems to come from the Old French *raspise*, a term meaning "sweet rose-colored wine."

S

Spinach

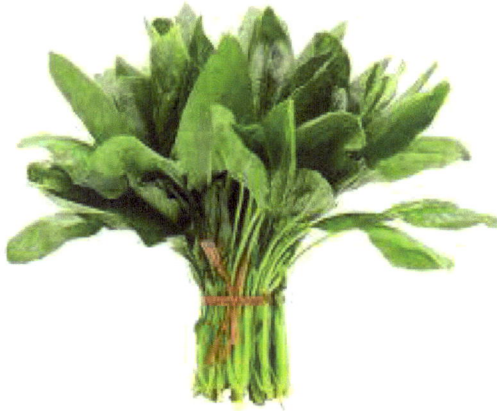

Spinach is best eaten fresh. It loses nutritional properties with each passing day.

T

Tomatoes

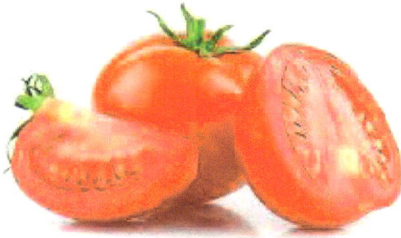

Because the **tomato** has seeds and grows from a
flowering plant botanically it is classed as a "fruit" not
a "vegetable."

U

Ugli

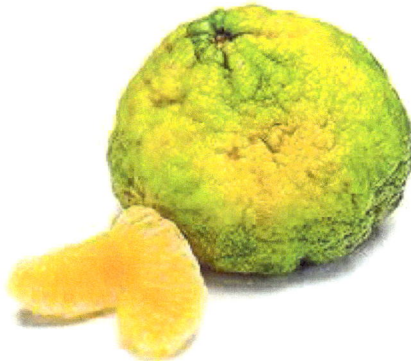

Ugli fruit is described as "a deliberate or accidental hybrid" of any mandarin orange and the grapefruit.

V

Vanilla Bean

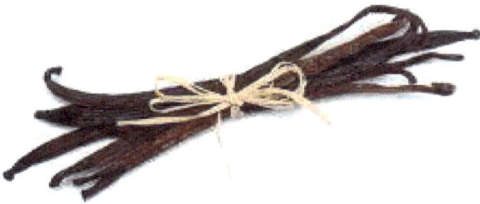

The flower that produces the **vanilla bean** lasts only
one day.

W

Watermelon

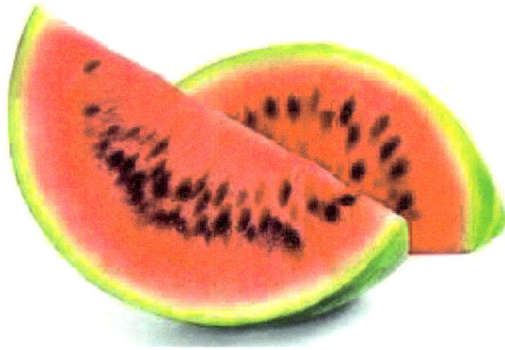

By weight, a **watermelon** contains about 6% sugar and 92% water.

X

Ximenia

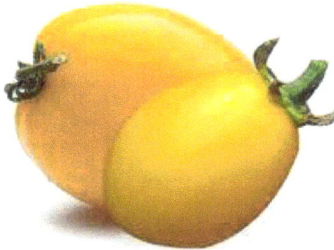

Ximenia Caffra fruit flesh is orange in color and edible with a bitter almond-like taste.

Y

Yams

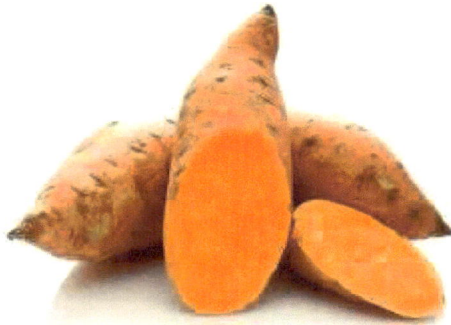

Yams should never be refrigerated until they're cooked.

Z

Zucchini

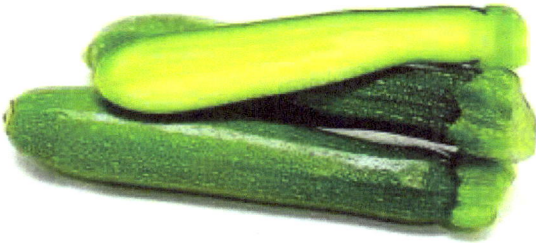

A **zucchini** has more potassium than a banana.

THE END....

Always FRESH!!!!

The Food Lord

Antonio Ford

www.ingramcontent.com/pod-product-compliance
Lightning Source LLC
Chambersburg PA
CBHW041215270326
41930CB00001B/35